Health Evidence Network synthesis report 44

Public health aspects of migrant health: a review of the evidence on health status for refugees and asylum seekers in the European Region

Hannah Bradby | Rachel Humphris | Dave Newall | Jenny Phillimore

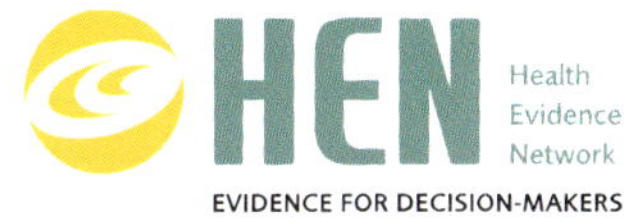

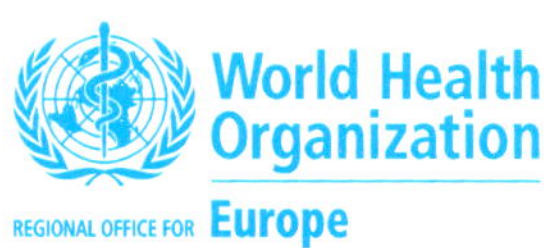

Abstract

Refugees and asylum seekers are defined in many ways but can be considered as those who did not make a voluntary choice to leave their country of origin and cannot return home in safety. Outcome data are limited and mostly focused on perinatal and mental health but do suggest significant levels of unmet need. This scoping review considered 72 studies where refugees and asylum seekers formed part or all of the population studied. Access to appropriate health care across the WHO European Region is very varied and is overwhelmingly shaped by legal frameworks and the regulation of the migration process. The need for improved communication with asylum seekers and coordinated action between agencies within and beyond the medical system is widely noted. Improved data to support intersectoral working to address the health care needs of asylum seekers and refugees are imperative.

Keywords
DELIVERY OF HEALTH CARE, EVIDENCE-BASED HEALTH CARE, HEALTH POLICY, REFUGEES, SOCIOECONOMIC FACTORS

Suggested citation

Bradby H, Humphris R, Newall D, Phillimore J. Public health aspects of migrant health: a review of the evidence on health status for refugees and asylum seekers in the European Region. Copenhagen: WHO Regional Office for Europe; 2015 (Health Evidence Network synthesis report 44).

Address requests about publications of the WHO Regional Office for Europe to:
    Publications
    WHO Regional Office for Europe
    UN City, Marmorvej 51
    DK-2100 Copenhagen Ø, Denmark
Alternatively, complete an online request form for documentation, health information, or for permission to quote or translate, on the Regional Office website (http://www.euro.who.int/pubrequest).

ISSN 2227-4316
ISBN 978 92 890 5110 1

© World Health Organization 2015

CONTENTS

ABBREVIATIONS

CIS	Commonwealth of Independent States
EU	European Union
HEN	Health Evidence Network
NGO	nongovernmental organization
UNHCR	United Nations High Commissioner for Refugees

CONTRIBUTORS

Authors

Hannah Bradby
Professor, Uppsala University, Uppsala, Sweden

Rachel Humphris
DPhil Student, Oxford University, Oxford, United Kingdom

Dave Newall
Independent consultant, Crewe, United Kingdom

Jenny Phillimore
Professor, University of Birmingham, Birmingham, United Kingdom

Collaborators

Magdalena Kania Lundholm
Post-doctoral research fellow, Uppsala University, Uppsala, Sweden

Amina Jama Mahmud
Post-doctoral researcher, Uppsala University, Uppsala, Sweden

Nando Sigona
Senior Lecturer, University of Birmingham, Birmingham, United Kingdom

External peer reviewers

Athena Linos
Professor of Medical School, Director of the Department of Hygiene, Epidemiology
and Medical Statistics, University of Athens, Athens, Greece

Tahereh Moradi
Associate Professor, Karolinska Institute, Stockholm, Sweden

Public Health Aspects of Migration and Health (PHAME) team

Santino Severoni, Coordinator
Rita Sá Machado
Rocío Zurriaga-Carda
Matteo Dembech
Sara Barragán-Montes
Grace M. Lassiter
Kate Langley

The PHAME team is part of the European Office for Investment for Health and Development, Division of Policy and Governance for Health and Well-being, WHO Regional Office for Europe.

Health Evidence Network (HEN) editorial team

Claudia Stein, Director
Tim Nguyen, Executive Editor
Ryoko Takahashi, Series Editor
Jane Ward, Copy Editor

The HEN editorial team is part of the Division of Information, Evidence, Research and Innovation, at the WHO Regional Office for Europe. HEN synthesis reports are commissioned works that are subjected to international peer review, and the contents are the responsibility of the authors. They do not necessarily reflect the official policies of the Regional Office.

FOREWORD

Zsuzsanna Jakab, WHO Regional Director for Europe

Migration is a high-priority topic on the policy agendas of most of the Member States in the WHO European Region. To address this priority, the WHO Regional Office for Europe established the Public Health Aspects of Migration in Europe (PHAME) project in 2012.

The main factors contributing to increased migration are natural and human-generated disasters, including social, economic and political instability.

The issues surrounding health and migration are important for a number of key reasons. They not only relate to the ethical implications of unequal access to health care but also are linked to (avoidable) costs to health systems and wider society. As a result, there is not only an ethical imperative to address issues of health and migration but also direct and indirect incentives, such as improved health, social cohesion, economic sustainability and political cooperation.

The lack of a single set of available data and the substantial variations from country to country mean that detecting Region-wide patterns or trends is difficult. The European Region encompasses a wide variety of natural environments and has a highly heterogeneous human geography. As a result, migration trends in the Region are highly complex, and differences between countries in the quality of data and collection methods compound the problems in any attempt to characterize them. Moreover, the collection and analysis of data require cooperation among migrants' countries of origin, transit and destination, and therefore collaboration beyond the boundaries of the European Region.

Evidence-based public health measures to mitigate the health implications of migration could save a significant number of lives and reduce suffering and ill health. They are also likely to be instrumental in effectively addressing growing health care costs and in preventing or mitigating the negative effects of migration on health systems and societies. Nevertheless, insufficient knowledge in many areas has hampered efforts towards more effective planning and implementation of effective strategies to address migration and health. A robust multidisciplinary scientific knowledge base is therefore an essential foundation for enhancing public health practices and policy development.

At its fifth meeting in July 2014, the European Advisory Committee on Health Research (EACHR) agreed to form a subcommittee on migration and health to review the PHAME strategic framework. EACHR recommended that the Secretariat commission three Health Evidence Network (HEN) synthesis reports tackling the challenges of three distinct migration groups: undocumented migrants, labour migrants, and refugees and asylum seekers. The subcommittee concluded that synthesizing and packaging existing evidence, rather than promoting new research, would be more useful for policy-makers.

This is one of the three commissioned reports, which focus on access to and delivery of health care for migrants. These will be the basis for identifying other aspects of health and migration that may be in need of additional research and evidence, and for the development of evidence-informed policies on migrant health and new approaches to improving migrants' health outcomes.

SUMMARY

The issue

Migration is considered a major social, political and public health challenge for the WHO European Region. The increase in numbers of refugees arriving in and travelling through the Region shows no sign of abating. Governments tend to distinguish between asylum seekers whose claims for refuge are under consideration and refugees whose claims are accepted. Asylum seekers and refugees often have differential access to welfare, particularly health services.

The synthesis question

The objective of this report is to synthesize research findings from a systematic review of available academic evidence and grey literature to address the following question. What policies and interventions work to improve health care access and delivery for asylum seekers and refugees in the European Region?

Types of evidence

A scoping review was undertaken of English language scholarly and grey literature and 72 studies were identified where refugees and asylum seekers formed part or all of the population studied.

Results

There was limited evidence on the health status of asylum seekers and refugees, with most focused on maternity and mental illness outcomes. Evidence of poorer mental health and perinatal outcomes for some refugees and asylum seekers suggests significant unmet need. However, the disadvantage is not consistent across all groups and cannot be generalized.

Access to health care is shaped by legal frameworks governing the rights of refugees and asylum seekers and by the regulation of the migration process. Other barriers in accessing health services include communication difficulties (e.g. lack of interpreters), cultural issues (e.g. gender preference for doctors), structural problems (e.g. transport) and bureaucratic barriers (e.g. social insurance systems). Access to specialist services can also be difficult. The nature and length of the asylum process plus the use of detention and dispersal can have a significant impact upon health outcomes. A good resettlement environment, including employment, family reunion, protection from discrimination and support for integration or repatriation, is associated with better health outcomes.

Policy considerations

Improved information and documentation is needed to support the design of national and international minimum standards and management strategies in the health and social care of refugees and asylum seekers. Policy options based on the evidence reviewed here are:

- improved access to services by removal of legal restrictions;

- provision of full health coverage for all pregnant women and for children regardless of immigration status;

- adoption of approaches to improve communications, such as provision of interpreters, good documentation for patients; and

- adjustment of health care provision to improve service utilization, for example longer appointment times, transport provision.

1. INTRODUCTION

1.1. Background

Migration is considered a major social, political and public health challenge for the WHO European Region; between 1990 and 2013, the number of international migrants worldwide rose by over 77 million and Europe had one of the largest growth rates of international migrants (1). Approximately half a million people sought asylum in Europe in 2013, a 32% increase since 2012, according to the United Nations High Commissioner for Refugees (UNHCR; Fig. 1 and 2) (2–4).[1] There is no evidence to suggest that numbers of refugees will fall in the near future; indeed, the ongoing "crisis" in the southern Mediterranean and Aegean suggests quite the opposite. In line with the framework of World Health Assembly Resolution 61.17 in 2008, the attention of Member States should be focused on ensuring equitable access to health promotion, disease prevention and care for migrants (5).

Refugees are formally owed protection, including access to health services, from their first country of registration for asylum. In practice, however, such rights may be routinely denied particularly at the asylum determination stage. Governments tend to distinguish between asylum seekers whose claims for refuge are under consideration and refugees whose claims have been accepted. Asylum seekers and refugees often have differential access to welfare, particularly health services. Delays in receipt of care may reflect local implementation limitations rather than national policies of provision (6). For refugees who do not or cannot declare themselves to the statutory authority, fear of detection may discourage access to health services. Undocumented or labour migrants may be forced migrants who are unable to claim asylum and, therefore, are not entitled to health care.

The rights to seek asylum vary across the WHO European Region, with certain countries within the Commonwealth of Independent States (CIS) refusing to recognize asylum claims from specific ethnic or national groups. Furthermore, the political will to support refugees, including providing health care, varies across the WHO European Region, with some governments notably disengaged.

---

[1] UNHCR European Region does not include Kazakhstan, Kyrgyzstan, Tajikistan, Turkmenistan or Uzbekistan.

Fig. 1. Refugees in Europe, December 2014

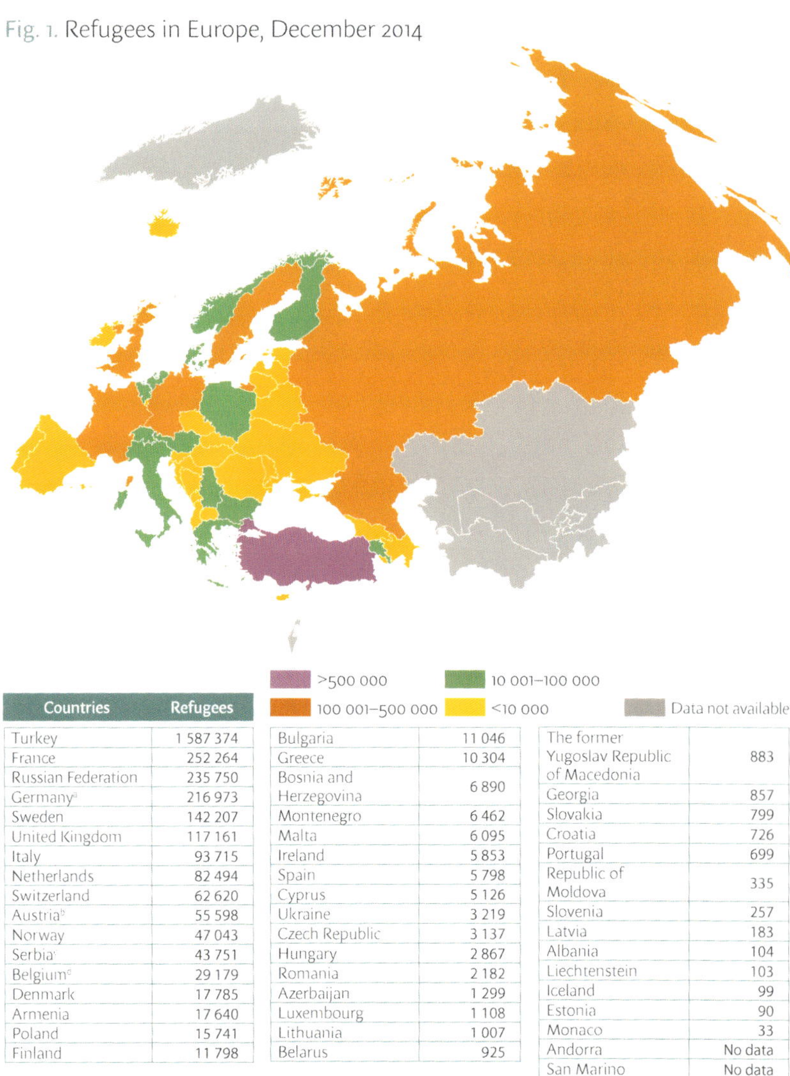

Countries	Refugees				
Turkey	1 587 374	Bulgaria	11 046	The former Yugoslav Republic of Macedonia	883
France	252 264	Greece	10 304	Georgia	857
Russian Federation	235 750	Bosnia and Herzegovina	6 890	Slovakia	799
Germany[a]	216 973	Montenegro	6 462	Croatia	726
Sweden	142 207	Malta	6 095	Portugal	699
United Kingdom	117 161	Ireland	5 853	Republic of Moldova	335
Italy	93 715	Spain	5 798	Slovenia	257
Netherlands	82 494	Cyprus	5 126	Latvia	183
Switzerland	62 620	Ukraine	3 219	Albania	104
Austria[b]	55 598	Czech Republic	3 137	Liechtenstein	103
Norway	47 043	Hungary	2 867	Iceland	99
Serbia[e]	43 751	Romania	2 182	Estonia	90
Belgium[c]	29 179	Azerbaijan	1 299	Monaco	33
Denmark	17 785	Luxembourg	1 108	Andorra	No data
Armenia	17 640	Lithuania	1 007	San Marino	No data
Poland	15 741	Belarus	925		
Finland	11 798				

[a] Figures reduced to align definitions; [b] Refers to the end of 2013; [d] Refers to mid-2014. [e] Serbia (and Kosovo (according to United Nations Security Council resolution 1244 (1999)).

Source: UNHCR, 2015 (3).

Fig. 2. Asylum and first-time asylum applicants in the European Union aggregated by citizenship, age and sex

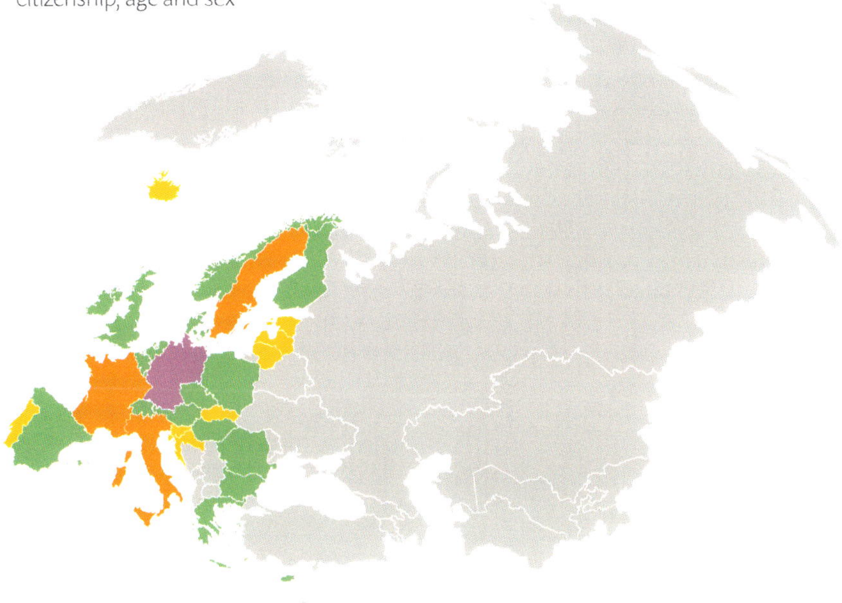

Countries	Asylum applicants				
Germany	202 815	Norway	11 480	Luxembourg	1 150
Sweden	81 325	Bulgaria	11 080	Croatia	450
Italy	64 625	Greece	9 435	Portugal	445
France	64 310	Poland	8 025	Lithuania	440
Hungary	42 775	Spain	5 615	Slovenia	385
United Kingdom	31 945	Finland	3 625	Latvia	375
Austria	28 065	Cyprus	1 745	Slovakia	330
Netherlands	24 535	Romania	1 545	Iceland	170
Switzerland	23 770	Ireland	1 450	Estonia	155
Belgium	22 850	Malta	1 350	Liechtenstein	75
Denmark	14 715	Czech Republic	1 155		

Source: Eurostat, 2015 (4).

This report responds to the synthesis question by reviewing the available evidence and examining which policies and interventions would work to improve accessibility and quality of health care delivery for asylum seekers and refugees.

A major problem in sourcing evidence is related to the wide variation in the definition and identification of refugees and asylum seekers used throughout the WHO European Region, as reflected in both scholarly and grey literature sourced (Annex 1). Not only do definitions vary, but their use is inconsistent. Migrants who are refugees and/or seeking asylum are a group whose definition is politically and administratively sensitive. What is meant by asylum seeker and refugee shifts, and the changing meanings have important political implications, including around access to health care (7). These changes in the process of "labelling" refugees have been informed by the interests of the nation state in controlling immigration (8) rather than by the goal of offering refuge and ensuring access to appropriate and equitable health care. Annex 2 summarizes the definitions of refugees, asylum seekers and migrants that can be found in the sourced literature. As a working definition for this analysis, the UNHCR describes a refugee as someone who did not make a conscious voluntary choice to leave their country of origin and cannot return home in safety.

1.2. Methodology

1.2.1. Sources for the review

Literature was found by searching the databases of the Cochrane Library, Web of Science, ProQuest, PubMed, ScienceDirect and the National Center for Biotechnology Information. Relevant scholarly papers and grey literature were identified that provided information on what is currently known about refugees and asylum seekers in terms of health status, access to and effectiveness of health services, and policies and interventions to reduce inequalities in health care delivery (6–77). Annex 1 outlines the databases searched and the review methodology.

Eurostat data were consulted for the European Economic Area and focused searches were undertaken to identify reports relevant for Armenia, Azerbaijan, Georgia, Kazakhstan, Kyrgyzstan, the Russian Federation, Tajikistan, Turkmenistan and Uzbekistan. Much of the material is not available in English.

1.2.2. Data extraction

Papers for inclusion were written in English, conducted in a WHO European Region Member State or included studies from that Region in the analysis of literature, were available as full text, and referred to refugees and asylum seekers explicitly in the disaggregated results. Only English literature was included due to limited resources. Because a limited number of papers addressed asylum seeker and refugee health as a unique group, a scoping review was conducted in which evidence was identified by a combination of keyword searching, focused Internet-based searching, searching of country-specific and sites specific to nongovernmental organizations (NGOs) and snowball-searching of reference lists. All sources were hand searched in full to identify further eligible studies. The objectives used for inclusion of relevant papers are:

- current demographic and geographical characteristics of asylum seekers and refugees in the WHO European Region with some detail of the social, political and legal living context;

- health status of asylum seekers and refugees, in particular with respect to areas of specific, major and re-emerging neglected diseases;

- delivery of health care to asylum seekers and refugees and their entitlement to it;

- quality of delivered health care in terms of accessibility, efficacy, appropriateness and equity;

- measures (health and economic indicators) used to assess asylum seekers and refugee status; or

- policies and communication strategies useful to improve health conditions and access to health care services of asylum seekers and refugees.

2. RESULTS

2.1. Health status

There is limited specific evidence on the health status of asylum seekers and refugees, making it hard to assess the impact of access difficulties. Evidence of poor health among refugees (9) is mostly confined to maternity and mental illness outcomes.

2.1.1. Maternity

Research tends not to disaggregate refugees and asylum seekers from other categories of migrant women, who in general have poorer birth outcomes than the general population after adjustment for age at delivery and parity (10). Reductions in the risks of these poor outcomes (including low birth weight, preterm delivery, perinatal mortality and congenital malformations) is associated with strong integration policies (10). Not all birth outcomes are poorer for vulnerable migrants (11), but there is evidence of serious unmet need among refugee and asylum-seeking women in terms of elevated perinatal mortality (12–16).

2.1.2. Mental health

Mental distress has higher prevalence among refugees compared with non-refugees (17), with a suggestion of greater risk for asylum seekers than for refugees (18). Risk factors associated with poor mental health include being a woman, older age, having experienced trauma, lacking social support and having more stress after migration (19). Consideration of conditions prior to and after migration show the influence of employment and education on health outcomes (20,21) and over the long term (22).

Unmet mental health needs among children, particularly unaccompanied minors (23) and those exposed to violence (24), suggests that their needs are not often distinguished from those of adult refugees (25). Despite the fragmentary baseline data, research shows that stable settlement and social support (24), including school participation, local friends and language proficiency, correlate with children's improved mental health (26).

2.2. Access to health care

Access to health care for refugees and asylum seekers is not only a problem of acute provision at initial reception. If people spend longer in a resettlement camp then care for chronic as well as acute health needs is required. Although some provision is specifically provided in detention or reception centres, refugees and asylum seekers across the WHO European Region are also accessing health care from the same clinics as the general population; consequently, adapting mainstream provision is crucial (6).

Access to health care varies across the WHO European Region in terms of legal entitlement and formal access regulations. Even where entitlement is established for formally resettled refugees (27), and regulations permit access, further impediments exist in terms of the organization of health care, limitations of health staff expertise as well as wider governance of migration.

There is scant evidence on the use of health care services by refugees and asylum seekers of different origins (19) or compared with non-migrant populations (28). Limited evidence exists for the underuse (29,30) and overuse (31,32) of services by refugees. Case study 1 outlines a report examining data that can be retrieved regarding use of health services by refugees and asylum seekers, and the problems of separating this group out from other migrants and other vulnerable groups in the general population (33). Difficulties in accessing general practice and an increased reliance on accident and emergency services for non-emergency treatment were identified, even though almost all the surveyed refugees were registered with a general practitioner. There was also evidence of late booking, poor antenatal care and poor pregnancy outcomes plus rates of mental health problems up to five times higher than the general population (33). It was concluded that improving access, particularly to primary care, is necessary (33). The low use of particular services or therapies by specific groups of asylum seekers or refugees also suggests inaccessibility (34). Impediments to access are described both in terms of the organization of health services and the wider context beyond the medical system (34).

2.2.1. Organization of services

Most services tend to evolve reactively rather than proactively, adapting to perceived or expressed needs of the population. Because numbers of asylum seekers and refugees in an area are difficult to predict, it is very hard for service providers to anticipate what the need is going to be in the near future. Services for asylum seekers and refugees can be considered as gateway services (facilitating access to mainstream services, assessment), core services (full primary care registration) and ancillary services (meeting additional specific health needs of refugees and asylum seekers) (35).

Case study 1. Determining access to care by vulnerable migrants

A report examining hidden needs of vulnerable groups in England collated data from sources that could inform policy on the health and health care needs of asylum seekers and refugees (33). Sources included the national census and other sources where numbers and health needs of refugees and asylum seekers might appear in official health and social care datasets; however, it was difficult to disaggregate asylum seekers and refugees from other migrants. In particular, it was difficult to assess their use of primary and secondary health services (with only country of birth being recorded in primary care, not in hospital databases) and mental health services for adults. By contrast, there was good capture of data for refugee and asylum-seeking children in need, in institutional care and requiring mental health services. Data for infectious diseases gave reasonable capture of migrants as a group, but poor disaggregation by type of migrant.

Access to primary care for asylum seekers and refugees can be promoted by collaboration between multidisciplinary staff; provision of no-cost or low-cost services, outreach services and free transport to and from appointments; longer clinic opening hours; patient advocacy; and use of gender-concordant providers (case study 2) (36,37). Practical support for patients to register, make appointments and attend services, for example through engaging interpreters to ensure clear explanations about unfamiliar clinical processes and treatments and timely management, is also effective in improving access (38). While NGOs supplement provision in some settings, their ability to provide continuity of care, refer to secondary care and use local resources such as general practitioners and nurses is less certain (39).

Case study 2. Adjustment of primary care in an area with a high proportion
of asylum seekers

Primary care teams in northern England with a high proportion of asylum
seekers adjusted service provision to improve access and quality of care in
several areas (37).

Linguistic needs include:
· documentation of the language and literacy level of all patients;
· provision of interpreters and communication with the patient in the language
  they understand best;
· longer appointment times to allow for interpretation and explanation; and
· simplified labelling of prescriptions for easier understanding.

Mobility of asylum seekers creates needs for:
· enhanced access to medical records, giving easier access for different agencies;
· provision of copies of written material for patients when they are referred
  to secondary care;
· regular contact with people registered with the practice to ensure that they
  are still in the area; and
· screening for homelessness.

Specific health service needs include:
· testing for HIV and sexually transmitted infections for high-risk groups;
· catch-up immunization for patients within 1 year; and
· screening for issues such as homelessness and a history of torture.

Staff expertise through:
· the provision of interpreters;
· enhanced cultural competency training; and
· enhanced intersectoral working.

To consolidate and sustain good practice, performance indicators that recognized
these services were developed at the Whitehouse Centre in Huddersfield,
United Kingdom.

2.2.2. Legal access

Beyond the health care system, wider legal and policy frameworks govern asylum and influence access to health care and who is responsible for care. Identification of the European Union (EU) Member State (plus Norway, Iceland, Liechtenstein and Switzerland) responsible for examination of an asylum claim in Europe is regulated by the Dublin Regulation, which came into force in July 2013. The Member State considered responsible for a particular person depends on the state by which the refugee enters the EU as well as family links. Where refugees are legally recognized and adequate health services exist, the legal status of an individual is the most important factor determining access to health care (40).

Across the WHO European Region, the ability of the state to provide health care for refugees and asylum seekers varies according to the development of health service infrastructure and the funding of health care for the general population. Where health infrastructure is underdeveloped or where refugees are not legally recognized, access to health care is inevitably poor. In countries near to a frontier or to a border with a conflict, the significant migrant flow, especially if made up of a high number of refugees, can mean that access to health care is very limited. These factors offer a particularly challenging combination in the CIS and central Asian states (41–45) as well as in the countries bordering the Mediterranean. In southern and eastern countries, there are no specialist mental health services for asylum seekers and refugees, while the use of accommodation centres (Germany, the Netherlands) and dispersal policies (United Kingdom) can disrupt access to, and appropriateness of, mainstream services (46,47). In addition, different routes to becoming a refugee and the structure of entitlements in a destination area can have a significant impact on health outcomes (case study 3) (40).

Legal entitlement does not guarantee access (2,27,48) and social insurance-based systems are particularly problematic for asylum seekers and refugees, since registration is more complex than in tax-funded systems (32).

2.2.3. Migration governance

Some features of the asylum process and the management of refugees have been identified not only as impeding access to health care but also as damaging well-being. An active dispersal policy can impede access to specialist health services (26,49,50) and may relocate refugees and asylum seekers to places where appropriate services have not been developed (23,49). Extended asylum procedures are associated with psychiatric disorders (51–54), particularly when involving detention (55) or the threat of detention or deportation. The harm increases with increasing length of detention (56) and persists longitudinally (57). Fear of jeopardizing an asylum application and social taboos can inhibit the disclosure of psychological symptoms (51). Even where leave to remain is granted, general stressors in the post-migration environment linked to social determinants of health, such as poverty, violence and threats, racism, acculturation stress and loss of family and friends (58,59), can damage health. Structural features, such as insecure asylum status, financial difficulties and discrimination affect children (60) and unaccompanied refugee minors (61).

Case study 3. The effects of structures of entitlement and routes of arrival on health and social care for pregnant women

A study of pregnant asylum-seeking and refugee women in Ireland illustrated the problems faced by refugees and asylum seekers in accessing health care, which can be significant to health outcomes (40).

Women did not receive the antenatal care to which they were entitled for a number of reasons:
- lack of language support;
- transport difficulties;
- childcare problems and having no accompanying partner or friend; and
- poor health and being too exhausted and stressed.

There were key differences in the support provided for the women depending on whether they were "programme refugees" who had arrived from Kosovo or those who had sought asylum upon arrival in Ireland. The widespread reporting of the war in Kosovo meant that the refugees were seen as victims, and so escaped the sense of disapproval that was reported by non-programme refugees. Provisions at the expense of the state were made for programme refugees that went some way to mitigate the anxiety and uncertainty common to all the refugee and asylum-seeking women; these included:
- reliable accommodation, and so some autonomy in relation to privacy and provision of their own food;
- individual access to translators;
- provision of an accompanying person for all antenatal and hospital visits; and
- transport provision, often taxi.

2.3. Barriers of communication, language and culture

Across the fragmentary available evidence, reduction of communication and language barriers is identified as key to improving access to services by migrants (62,63) and provision of services by health professionals (64–66). Lack of a common language between staff and patient is associated with decreased symptom reporting and fewer referrals to secondary and specialist care (67). Without adequate communication, refugees and asylum seekers receive poor care (68,69) and their access to wider support is hindered (70).

While a common language is crucial, "culturally competent" services should offer more than just minimal communication. A health care professional should be able to explain the host country's system of health care (71), as well as grasping the political situation of the migrant's country of origin and being aware of the specific diseases common in the countries of origin (72). Awareness of the legal context, knowledge of how refugee status influences health and well-developed skills in asking delicate questions about traumatic events are also key requirements (72). In clinical settings where people from multiple linguistic and national groups are treated, detailed knowledge of all the potential backgrounds may be unrealistic (12). Nonetheless, "migrant-friendly" approaches can use use telephone interpreting, face-to-face interpreting, intercultural mediation and supportive written information to improve clinical communication for both providers and patients (65).

Health and welfare services are constructed around a particular biomedical definition of good health; where this differs from how refugees conceptualize health, appropriate care may be very hard to achieve (73). Refugees' conceptions of health can differ from those of professionals (74) in that terms of happiness can be considered by the refugee as being both a prerequisite for and an indication of healthiness (75); consequently, life in exile, characterized by poverty and discrimination, may never be considered healthy (76). These ambiguous expectations mean that even asylum seekers with adequate linguistic knowledge may lack medical terminology or ways of communicating symptoms.

Health services are often designed with the assumption that patients have specific cultural skills and communication competencies (12). While the routes used by asylum seekers and refugees to solve health problems suggest agency and ingenuity (77), they may nonetheless lack the skills to make the most of a health service, particularly when seeking care from multiple agencies. To respond adequately to the health and the social care needs of refugees and asylum seekers, intersectoral communication and organization by professionals is essential (case study 2) (36). Nongovernmental and voluntary agencies often bridge gaps of communication and access for refugees and asylum seekers, but their ability to refer widely enough and to provide continuity of care is limited.

3. DISCUSSION

3.1. Strengths and limitations of the review

The scholarly literature was dominated by research from the United Kingdom, the Netherlands and Scandinavia, which limits the generalizability of findings to other settings. There was wide variation in the definitions used for asylum seeker and refugee in different settings and across research and reports (Annex 2), and this made it hard to ensure that the same population was being described. In addition, many studies refer to migrants as a whole or to vulnerable groups that include asylum seekers and refugees. Where findings suggest a contrast in prevalence or rates of access, this may reflect methodological differences. For example, migrants may be compared in surveys with the host country's general population or the host country's non-migrant population from similar ethnic groups. In some studies, migrant population may be defined with respect to cross-border movement, while in others migrants are defined based on their reported ethnicity. Discrepancies in response rates may also reflect heterogeneity within migrant groups. The evidence about the effectiveness and quality of health care for asylum seekers and refugees is also difficult to assess given the diversity of health care organization within national and regional boundaries. The lack of common strategies for health care management of refugees is apparent in the fragmented nature of the identified data.

Even though evidence is limited, there are examples of successful intersectoral interventions that foster integration and promote communication between and beyond medical agencies, focused on migrants' assessment of their needs. In addition, some barriers to accessing health care are consistently highlighted in the literature, including legal and structural impediments, absence of language provision, cultural communication and expectations, and lack of clear guidance on entitlement (32). There are also examples of good practice (case studies 2 and 3) that can act as models.

3.2. Access to care and health status

Definition and identification of refugees and asylum seekers is widely diverse and inconsistent across the WHO European Region, implying both political sensitivities and specific challenges, including around access to health care (7). It should also be noted that the Region includes many refugee-producing countries as well as refugee-receiving countries. Internally displaced people and the growing number of stateless people must also be considered within the Region, although the published academic literature does not address this. Creation of a consistent labelling system for asylum seekers and refugees in the WHO European Region would simplify progress on ensuring access to appropriate and equitable health care for this group.

There is limited evidence on the health status of asylum seekers and refugees. Research tends to assume that asylum seekers and refugees have specific and elevated health needs, despite the lack of systematic evidence. Evidence of poor health among refugees (9) is mostly confined to maternity and mental illness outcomes, with little clear data on infectious diseases and chronic conditions in this particular group.

Access to health care varies across the WHO European Region and within national boundaries, particularly where individuals are dispersed away from large cities where provision is often focused in terms of legal entitlement and formal access regulations. Where state systems are ineffective or not accessible, reliance on NGOs to bridge gaps in communication and access is high. Legal status determines the resources that refugees and asylum seekers can access. An extended process of asylum determination that has involved detention, social isolation and poverty is detrimental to health. Effective integration policies and socioeconomic security reduce health risk and should be encouraged. Although particular barriers can be identified in terms of prevention of uptake of health care services, the effects of the overall configuration of services is less often assessed. Practical support for patients to register, make appointments and attend services through engaging interpreters to ensure clear explanations about unfamiliar clinical processes and treatments is effective in improving access (33,37). Primary health care often plays a gatekeeping role in accessing other services, which makes this a crucial site for appropriate linguistic and cultural interpretation (37). Apart from specific actions to improve communications, such as interpreter services, advocacy support and strong integration programmes can help asylum seekers and refugees to access health care and could mitigate long-term health problems (37).

With clear indications that the numbers of asylum seekers undergoing perilous and traumatic journeys is increasing, the health impacts of these processes should be studied. The challenge of acquiring quality data to compare the health needs of refugees and asylum seekers with other sections of the population, plus identifying their specific structural and socioeconomic context, is considerable. Health penalties are consistently found, for example in terms of poorer mental health and perinatal outcomes, but the evidence is neither consistent nor generalizable.

Potential difficulties in accessing health care for refugees or asylum seekers can be summarized as follows:

- documentation: literacy and language issues may act as barriers to engaging in systems requiring high levels of documentation;

- confusion about entitlement: differential entitlements associated with varying migrant status enhances confusion for both health seeker and health professional, and professionals to refuse services;

- organization of health services in conjunction with immigration services: can mean that specialist services rather than mainstream ones must be used;

- geographic issues: health services in capital cities away from refugee reception or detention centres and a lack of affordable transport links;

- funding structures: unemployed and/or poor asylum seekers and refugees may lack the documentation and/or resources to cover costs in a social insurance system; and

- informal payments: unemployed and/or poor asylum seekers and refugees may lack resources to cover costs.

3.3. Policy options and implications

A number of policy options can be considered based on this review. These relate both to policies to improve access to health care for asylum seekers and refugees and to steps to gather data that will enable policy-makers to make evidence-informed decisions.

Practical support to facilitate access to services could be provided through:

- removal of any legal restrictions on access to health care for asylum seekers and refugees;

- extension of full health care coverage to all children regardless of their immigration status;

- extension of full health care coverage to all pregnant women regardless of their immigration status with assistance at delivery and parity; and

- coordinated action between agencies within and beyond the medical system, including integration of housing, employment and education.

Linguistic barriers to quality health care could be addressed through:

- adoption of an intersectoral approach to the provision and distribution of health information in a range of languages;
- provision of professional interpreters, free of cost to the patient and health professional;
- provision of clear labelling for prescriptions with specific consideration for the language of the patient; and
- documentation of language and literacy levels of patients.

Utilization of services, particularly primary care, could be improved, with:

- provision of technical support for registering and making appointments, including language support and patient advocacy services;
- provision of free transport to and from appointments;
- longer appointment times, thus allowing for interpretation and explanation;
- provision of flexible opening hours and appointment times;
- gender specific requests being met and respected;
- development and delivery of quality training for professionals, considering cultural sensitivity in health care delivery; and
- increased awareness among health professionals of mental health issues for refugees and asylum seekers, particularly minors.

The evidence on health issues for refugees and asylum seekers could be strengthened by developing information and monitoring systems to promote:

- comparative work across subsections of migrant and non-migrant populations, considering using the concept of "recency of arrival" to cut across different migrant statuses at this entry stage;
- coordination of data across governmental and nongovernmental agencies;
- examination of the health effects of different phases of the asylum process;
- assessment of the long-term health impacts of initiatives relating to integration in housing, employment and education;

- understanding of the correlation between integration policy and good health outcomes in maternity and mental health;

- development of non-stigmatizing concepts for research and monitoring; and

- address of migrants' own priorities and where these may be at odds with those of professionals.

4. CONCLUSIONS

Migration is a major social, political and public health challenge for the WHO European Region and policy-makers will need to develop specific and coherent policies addressing the health needs of all migrants, including asylum seekers and refugees. The lack of common strategies for the health care management of refugees is apparent in the fragmented nature of data described here. Health penalties are consistently found in terms of poorer mental health and perinatal outcomes, but the evidence is neither consistent nor generalizable. The variation in how countries define asylum seekers and refugees and in how health care is provided at point of entry and at final destination also make it harder to draw generalized evidence-based conclusions. However, even though evidence is limited, there are examples of successful intersectoral interventions that foster integration and promote communication between and beyond medical agencies. Legal and structural impediments as well as uncertainties in communication, expectation and entitlement are described as the main barriers for this population to access health care. A lack of specialized maternal and mental health services is noted. Improving the collection of quality of data, prioritizing measurement and mapping of good practices and encouraging research to underpin the development of minimum standards in health and social care of refugees all actions that should be reinforced.

REFERENCES

1. International migration report 2013. New York: United Nations, Department of Economic and Social Affairs; 2013 (http://www.un.org/en/development/desa/population/migration/publications/wallchart/docs/wallchart2013.pdf, accessed 29 July 2015).

2. UNHCR Global Report 2013: Europe regional summary. Geneva: United Nations High Commissioner for Refugees; 2013 (http://www.unhcr.org/539809e10.html, accessed 29 July 2015).

3. UNHCR 2015 regional operations profile: Europe. Geneva: United Nations High Commissioner for Refugees; 2015 (http://www.unhcr.org/pages/4a02d9346.html, accessed 28 July 2015).

4. Asylum and first time asylum applicants by citizenship, age and sex, annual aggregated data. Luxembourg: Eurostat, 2015.

5. Sixty-first World Health Assembly. Health of migrants. Geneva: World Health Organization; 2008 (WHA61.17) (http://apps.who.int/gb/ebwha/pdf_files/A61/A61_R17-en.pdf, accessed 21 July 2015).

6. Ager A. Health and forced migration. In: Fiddian-Qasmiyeh E, Loescher G, Long K, Sigona N, editors. The Oxford handbook of refugee and forced migration studies. Oxford: Oxford University Press; 2014.

7. Zetter R. Labelling refugees: forming and transforming a bureaucratic identity. J Refug Stud. 1991;4(1):39–62.

8. Zetter R. More labels, fewer refugees: remaking the refugee label in an era of globalization. J Refug Stud. 2007;20(2):172–92.

9. Wangdahl J, Lytsy P, Martensson L, Westerling R. Health literacy among refugees in Sweden: a cross-sectional study. BMC Public Health. 2014;14:1030.

10. Bollini P, Pampallona S, Wanner P, Kupelnick B. Pregnancy outcome of migrant women and integration policy: a systematic review of the international literature. Soc Sci Med. 2009;68(3):452–61.

11. Gagnon AJ, Zimbeck M, Zeitlin J. Migration to western industrialised countries and perinatal health: a systematic review. Soc Sci Med. 2009;69(6):934–46.

12. Phillimore J. Delivering maternity services in an era of superdiversity: the challenges of novelty and newness. Ethn Racial Stud. 2015;38(4):568–82.

13. Lalchandani S, MacQuillan K, Sheil O. Obstetric profiles and pregnancy outcomes of immigrant women with refugee status. Ir Med J. 2001;94(3):79–80.

14. Råssjö EB, Byrskog U, Samir R, Klingberg-Allvin M. Somali women's use of maternity health services and the outcome of their pregnancies: a descriptive study comparing Somali immigrants with native-born Swedish women. Sex Reprod Health. 2013;4(3):99–106.

15. Small R, Gagnon A, Gissler M, Zeitlin J, Bennis M, Glazier R et al. Somali women and their pregnancy outcomes postmigration: data from six receiving countries. BJOG Int J Obstet Gynaecol. 2008;115(13):1630–40.

16. Lewis G. Saving mothers' lives: reviewing maternal deaths to make motherhood safer, 2003–2005. London: Confidential Enquiry into Maternal and Child Health; 2007.

17. Porter M, Haslam N. Predisplacement and postdisplacement factors associated with mental health of refugees and internally displaced persons: a meta-analysis. JAMA. 2005;294(5):602–12.

18. Fazel M, Wheeler J, Danesh J. Prevalence of serious mental disorder in 7000 refugees resettled in western countries: a systematic review. Lancet. 2005;365(9467):1309–14.

19. Gerritsen AAM, Bramsen I, Devillé W, van Willigen LHM, Hovens JE, van der Ploeg HM. Use of health care services by Afghan, Iranian, and Somali refugees and asylum seekers living in the Netherlands. Eur J Public Health. 2006;16(4):394–9.

20. Hermansson A-C, Timpka T, Thyberg M. The long-term impact of torture on the mental health of war-wounded refugees: findings and implications for nursing programmes. Scand J Caring Sci. 2003;17(4):317–24.

21. Masmas TN, Møller E, Buhmannr C, Bunch V, Jensen JH, Hansen TN et al. Asylum seekers in Denmark: a study of health status and grade of traumatization of newly arrived asylum seekers. Torture. 2008;18(2):77–86.

22. Roth G, Ekblad S. A longitudinal perspective on depression and sense of coherence in a sample of mass-evacuated adults from Kosovo. J Nerv Ment Dis. 2006;194(5):378–81.

23. Bean TM, Eurelings-Bontekoe E, Spinhoven P. Course and predictors of mental health of unaccompanied refugee minors in the Netherlands: one year follow-up. Soc Sci Med. 2007;64(6):1204–15.

24. Fazel M, Reed RV, Panter-Brick C, Stein A. Mental health of displaced and refugee children resettled in high-income countries: risk and protective factors. Lancet. 2012;379(9812):266–82.

25. Derluyn I, Broekaert E. Unaccompanied refugee children and adolescents: the glaring contrast between a legal and a psychological perspective. Int J Law Psychiatry. 2008;31(4):319–30.

26. Montgomery E. Trauma, exile and mental health in young refugees. Acta Psychiatr Scand. 2011;124:1–46.

27. Peiro MJ, Benedict R. Migration health: better health for all in Europe. Brussels: International Organization for Migration; 2009 (http://www.migrant-health-europe.org/files/AMAC%20Public%20Report.pdf, accessed 18 July 2015).

28. Alkahtani S, Cherrill J, Millward C, Grayson K, Hilliam R, Sammons H et al. Access to medicines by child refugees in the East Midlands region of England: a cross-sectional study. BMJ Open. 2014;4(12):e006421.

29. Brendler-Lindqvist M, Norredam M, Hjern A. Duration of residence and psychotropic drug use in recently settled refugees in Sweden: a register-based study. Int J Equity Health. 2014;13:122.

30. Gernaat HBPE, Malwand AD, Laban CJ, Komproe I, de Jong JTVM. Many psychiatric disorders in Afghan refugees with residential status in Drenthe, especially depressive disorder and post-traumatic stress disorder. Ned Tijdschr Geneeskd. 2002;146(24):1127–31.

31. Toar M, O'Brien KK, Fahey T. Comparison of self-reported health and healthcare utilisation between asylum seekers and refugees: an observational study. BMC Public Health. 2009;9:214.

32. Collantes S. Are undocumented migrants and asylum seekers entitled to access health care in the EU? A comparative overview in 16 countries. Madrid: HUMA Network; 2011 (http://www.epim.info/wp-content/uploads/2011/02/HUMA-Publication-Comparative-Overview-16-Countries-2010.pdf, accessed 16 July 2015).

33. Aspinall PJ. Hidden needs. Identifying key vulnerable groups in data collections: vulnerable migrants, gypsies and travellers, homeless people, and sex workers. Brighton: Centre for Health Services Studies, University of Kent; 2014 (https://www.gov.uk/government/uploads/system/uploads/attachment_data/file/287805/vulnerable_groups_data_collections.pdf, accessed 29 July 2015).

34. Robertson E, Johansson S E. Use of complementary, non-pharmacological pain reduction methods during childbirth among foreign-born and Swedish-born women. Midwifery. 2010;26(4):442–9.

35. Feldman R. Primary health care for refugees and asylum seekers: a review of the literature and a framework for services. Public Health. 2006;120:809–16.

36. Joshi C, Russell G, Cheng I-H, Kay M, Pottie K, Alston M et al. A narrative synthesis of the impact of primary health care delivery models for refugees in resettlement countries on access, quality and coordination. Int J Equity Health. 2013;12:88.

37. Eling J. Asylum seeker, refugee and vulnerable migrant services. Mapping and best practice report and recommendations. London: Maternity Action; 2010 (http://www.maternityaction.org.uk/sitebuildercontent/sitebuilderfiles/new_refugee_and_migrant_services_mapping_and_best_practice_reportv3.pdf, accessed 29 July 2015).

38. Cheng I-H, Drillich A, Schattner P. Refugee experiences of general practice in countries of resettlement: a literature review. Br J Gen Pract J R Coll Gen Pract. 2015;65(632):e171–6.

39. Hardy JN. Underfunding of primary care in deprived areas affects everyone. BMJ. 2006;332(7535):236.

40. Kennedy P, Murphy-Lawless J. The maternity care needs of refugee and asylum seeking women in Ireland. Fem Rev. 2003;(73):39–53.

41. Regamey A, Booth K, McKune S. Kazakhstan/Kyrgyzstan: exploitation of migrant workers, protection denied to asylum seekers and refugees. Paris: International Federation for Human Rights; 2009 (http://www2.ohchr.org/english/bodies/cerd/docs/ngos/FIDH_Kazakhstan_76.pdf, accessed 16 July 2015).

42. Mladovsky P, Ingleby D, Rechel B. Good practices in migrant health: the European experience. Clin Med. 2012;12(3):248–52.

43. Mladovsky P, Rechel B, Ingleby D, McKee M. Responding to diversity: an exploratory study of migrant health policies in Europe. Health Policy. 2012;105(1):1–9.

44. UNHCR Global Report 2007: Central Asia section. Geneva: United Nations High Commissioner for Refugees; 2007 (http://www.unhcr.org/48490d192.html, accessed 29 July 2015).

45. Kazakhstan fact sheet. Geneva: United Nations High Commissioner for Refugees; 2014 (http://www.unhcr.org/500016019.html, accessed 17 July 2015).

46. Watters C, Ingleby D. Locations of care: meeting the mental health and social care needs of refugees in Europe. Int J Law Psychiatry. 2004;27:549–70.

47. Ingleby D, Watters C. Mental health and social care for asylum seekers and refugees. In: Ingleby D, editor. Forced migration and mental health. New York: Springer; 2005:193–212 (http://link.springer.com/chapter/10.1007/0-387-22693-1_12, accessed 15 May 2015).

48. Health of migrants: the way forward: report of a global consultation, Madrid, Spain, 3–5 March 2010. Geneva: World Health Organization; 2010 (http://www.who.int/hac/events/consultation_report_health_migrants_colour_web.pdf, accessed 15 July 2015).

49. Creighton S, Sethi G, Edwards SG, Miller R. Dispersal of HIV positive asylum seekers: national survey of UK healthcare providers. BMJ. 2004;329(7461):322–3.

50. Hogan H. Meeting health needs of asylum seekers. White paper will make access to health care more difficult. BMJ. 1999;318(7184):671.

51. Collins CH, Zimmerman C, Howard LM. Refugee, asylum seeker, immigrant women and postnatal depression: rates and risk factors. Arch Womens Ment Health. 2011;14(1):3–11.

52. Laban CJ, Gernaat H, Komproe IH, Schreuders BA, de Jong J. Impact of a long asylum procedure on the prevalence of psychiatric disorders in Iraqi asylum seekers in the Netherlands. J Nerv Ment Dis. 2004;192(12):843–51.

53. Staehr MA, Munk-Andersen E. Suicide and suicidal behavior among asylum seekers in Denmark during the period 2001–2003. A retrospective study. Ugeskr Laeger. 2006;168(17):1650–3.

54. Hallas P, Hansen AR, Stæhr MA, Munk-Andersen E, Jorgensen HL. Length of stay in asylum centres and mental health in asylum seekers: a retrospective study from Denmark. BMC Public Health. 2007;7(1):288.

55. Cohen J. Safe in our hands?: A study of suicide and self-harm in asylum seekers. J Forensic Leg Med. 2008;15(4):235–44.

56. Steel Z, Silove D, Brooks R, Momartin S, Alzuhairi B, Susljik INA. Impact of immigration detention and temporary protection on the mental health of refugees. Br J Psychiatry. 2006;188(1):58–64.

57. Robjant K, Hassan R, Katona C. Mental health implications of detaining asylum seekers: systematic review. Br J Psychiatry. 2009;194(4):306–12.

58. Blight KJ, Ekblad S, Lindencrona F, Shahnavaz S. Promoting mental health and preventing mental disorder among refugees in western countries. Int J Ment Health Promot. 2009;11(1):32–44.

59. Lindencrona F, Ekblad S. Refugee resettlement programmes as potential mental health promoting settings? A qualitative study of resettlement staff's constructions of refugees' mental health in everyday episodes. Int J Migr Health Soc Care. 2006;2(1):48–62.

60. Heptinstall E, Sethna V, Taylor E. PTSD and depression in refugee children. Eur Child Adolesc Psychiatry. 2004;13(6):373–80.

61. Ramel B, Taljemark J, Lindgren A, Johansson BA. Overrepresentation of unaccompanied refugee minors in inpatient psychiatric care. SpringerPlus. 2015;4:131.

62. Straus L, McEwen A, Hussein FM. Somali women's experience of childbirth in the UK: perspectives from Somali health workers. Midwifery. 2009;25(2):181–6.

63. O'Donnell CA, Higgins M, Chauhan R, Mullen K. "They think we're OK and we know we're not." A qualitative study of asylum seekers' access, knowledge and views to health care in the UK. BMC Health Serv Res. 2007;7:75.

64. Fatahi N, Nordholm L, Mattsson B, Hellström M. Experiences of Kurdish war-wounded refugees in communication with Swedish authorities through interpreter. Patient Educ Couns. 2010;78(2):160–5.

65. Novak-Zezula S, Schulze B, Karl-Trummer U, Krajic K, Pelikan JM. Improving interpreting in clinical communication: models of feasible practice from the European project "Migrant-friendly Hospitals". Divers Health Soc Care. 2005;2(3):223–32.

66. Ochieng BMN. Black African migrants: the barriers with accessing and utilizing health promotion services in the UK. Eur J Public Health. 2013;23(2):265–9.

67. Bischoff A, Bovier PA, Isah R, Françoise G, Ariel E, Louis L. Language barriers between nurses and asylum seekers: their impact on symptom reporting and referral. Soc Sci Med. 2003;57(3):503–12.

68. Kurth E, Jaeger FN, Zemp E, Tschudin S, Bischoff A. Reproductive health care for asylum-seeking women: a challenge for health professionals. BMC Public Health. 2010;10:659.

69. Bulman KH, McCourt C. Somali refugee women's experiences of maternity care in west London: a case study. Crit Public Health. 2002;12(4):365–80.

70. Byrskog U, Olsson P, Essen B, Allvin M-K. Being a bridge: Swedish antenatal care midwives' encounters with Somali-born women and questions of violence; a qualitative study. BMC Pregn Childbirth. 2015;15:1.

71. Suurmond J, Seeleman C, Rupp I, Goosen S, Stronks K. Cultural competence among nurse practitioners working with asylum seekers. Nurse Educ Today. 2010;30(8):821–6.

72. Suurmond J, Rupp I, Seeleman C, Goosen S, Stronks K. The first contacts between healthcare providers and newly-arrived asylum seekers: a qualitative study about which issues need to be addressed. Public Health. 2013;127(7):668–73.

73. Grønseth AS. Tamil refugees in pain: challenging solidarity in the Norwegian welfare state. J Ethn Migr Stud. 2011;37(2):315–32.

74. Zepinic V, Bogic M, Priebe S. Refugees' views of the effectiveness of support provided by their host countries. Eur J Psychotraumatol. 2012;3:10. (http://www.ncbi.nlm.nih.gov/pmc/articles/PMC3480961/, accessed 29 July 2015).

75. Papadopoulos I, Lees S, Lay M, Gebrehiwot A. Ethiopian refugees in the UK: migration, adaptation and settlement experiences and their relevance to health. Ethn Health. 2004;9(1):55–73.

76. Svenberg K, Skott C, Lepp M. Ambiguous expectations and reduced confidence: experience of Somali refugees encountering Swedish Health Care. J Refug Stud. 2011;fer026:1–16 (http://www.narhalsan.se/upload/FoUU-PVG/Aktuellt/KristianSvenberg_Hermeneutik.pdf, accessed 29 July 2015).

77. Bhatia R, Wallace P. Experiences of refugees and asylum seekers in general practice: a qualitative study. BMC Fam Pract. 2007;8:48.

ANNEX 1. SEARCH STRATEGY

Databases

The search used the databases of the Cochrane Library, Web of Science, ProQuest, PubMed, ScienceDirect and the National Center for Biotechnology Information. Eurostat data was consulted for the European Economic Area.

Search terms

TOPIC: (migrant* or migration or immigra* or foreign* or (minority near groups) or refuge* or asylum) AND TOPIC: (policy or policies or intervention* or law or laws or program* or service* or reform* or access* or planning or delivery) AND TOPIC: (health or medical)

ANNEX 2. DEFINITIONS OF REFUGEES, ASYLUM SEEKERS AND MIGRANTS IN THE LITERATURE

The term asylum seeker might be expected to denote those who have not (or not yet) been given international protection. The term refugee should then cover all those who are seeking asylum, regardless of the recognition of their claim – an argument frequently made by organizations such as the Refugee Council. "Refugees" may refer to all those fleeing persecution or only to those with the legal right to remain in the country of refuge (1). However, the research described in this report (a) used the term "refugee" to denote "refugee" and "asylum seeker" (2,3), (b) used the terms "refugee" and "asylum seeker" interchangeably (4–6), or (c) conflated the two (7), since the line between refugee and migrant is "very fuzzy" (8).

From a policy perspective, many governments define asylum seekers as those awaiting a decision on their claim for asylum. In this context, refugees are defined as those who have been successful in their claim, and those who are unsuccessful are defined as failed asylum seekers. "Failed asylum seekers" may be able to appeal the decision and make a fresh claim. In so doing, their legal right to claim health care changes in certain countries.

In some papers, no definition of the terms is offered (9,10). Some of the papers cited in this review focus on all asylum seekers or on the total immigrant population, which may include some refugees and asylum seekers where they are explicitly disaggregated in results.

Few studies acknowledged that asylum seekers and refugees are a heterogeneous group with widely differing experiences, backgrounds, health needs and health behaviours (11). Similarly, a descriptive historical and political account of the specific situation of movement and reception of asylum seekers was rare (12–14).

Reference to the legal definition of asylum seekers as those exercising their right to claim asylum, as defined by the Universal Declaration of Human Rights, is common (3,15–21). Similarly, refugee status, as defined by the United Nations Convention relating to the Status of Refugees is regularly noted (22–24).

The United Nations High Commissioner for Refugees (UNHCR) describes a "migrant" as someone who makes a conscious, voluntary choice to leave their country of origin and who, when they want to, can return home in safety, whereas refugees do not have this option (16). Few papers address the conceptual problems of defining refugees and asylum seekers (17). Given the lack of clarity in distinguishing between refugees and asylum seekers, it is not surprising that only one study systematically sought differences in disease prevalence between refugees and asylum seekers (14).

References

1. Cohen J. Safe in our hands?: A study of suicide and self-harm in asylum seekers. J Forensic Leg Med. 2008;15(4):235–44.

2. Bhatia R, Wallace P. Experiences of refugees and asylum seekers in general practice: a qualitative study. BMC Fam Pract. 2007;8:48.

3. Alkahtani S, Cherrill J, Millward C, Grayson K, Hilliam R, Sammons H et al. Access to medicines by child refugees in the East Midlands region of England: a cross-sectional study. BMJ Open. 2014;4(12):e006421.

4. Bischoff A, Bovier PA, Isah R, Françoise G, Ariel E, Louis L. Language barriers between nurses and asylum seekers: their impact on symptom reporting and referral. Soc Sci Med. 2003;57(3):503–12.

5. Burnett A, Peel M. Asylum seekers and refugees in Britain: health needs of asylum seekers and refugees. BMJ. 2001;322:544–7.

6. Cheng I-H, Drillich A, Schattner P. Refugee experiences of general practice in countries of resettlement: a literature review. Br J Gen Pract J R Coll Gen Pract. 2015;65(632):e171–6.

7. Başoğlu M, Ekblad S, Bäärnhielm S, Livanou M. Cognitive-behavioral treatment of tortured asylum seekers: a case study. J Anxiety Disord. 2004;18(3):357–69.

8. Derluyn I, Mels C, Broekaert E. Mental health problems in separated refugee adolescents. J Adolesc Health. 2009;44(3):291–7.

9. O'Donnell CA, Higgins M, Chauhan R, Mullen K. Asylum seekers' expectations of and trust in general practice: a qualitative study. Br J Gen Pract J R Coll Gen Pract. 2008;58(557):e1–11.

10. Redman EA, Reay HJ, Jones L, Roberts RJ. Self-reported health problems of asylum seekers and their understanding of the national health service: a pilot study. Public Health. 2011;125(3):142–4.

11. Suurmond J, Rupp I, Seeleman C, Goosen S, Stronks K. The first contacts between healthcare providers and newly-arrived asylum seekers: a qualitative study about which issues need to be addressed. Public Health. 2013;127(7):668–73.

12. Papadopoulos I, Lees S, Lay M, Gebrehiwot A. Ethiopian refugees in the UK: migration, adaptation and settlement experiences and their relevance to health. Ethn Health. 2004;9(1):55–73.

13. O'Donnell CA, Higgins M, Chauhan R, Mullen K. "They think we're OK and we know we're not." A qualitative study of asylum seekers' access, knowledge and views to health care in the UK. BMC Health Serv Res. 2007;7:75.

14. Gerritsen AA, Bramsen I, Devillé W, van Willigen LH, Hovens JE, van der Ploeg HM. Physical and mental health of Afghan, Iranian and Somali asylum seekers and refugees living in the Netherlands. Soc Psychiatry Psychiatr Epidemiol. 2006;41(1):18–26.

15. Norredam M, Mygind A, Krasnik A. Access to health care for asylum seekers in the European Union: a comparative study of country policies. Eur J Public Health. 2006;16(3):285–9.

16. Reeves M, de Wildt G, Murshali H, Williams P, Gill P, Kralj L et al. Access to health care for people seeking asylum in the UK. Br J Gen Pract. 2006;56(525):306–8.

17. Taylor K. Asylum seekers, refugees, and the politics of access to health care: a UK perspective. Br J Gen Pract. 2009;59(567):765–72.

18. Pieper H-O, Clerkin P, MacFarlane A. The impact of direct provision accommodation for asylum seekers on organisation and delivery of local primary care and social care services: a case study. BMC Fam Pract. 2011;12:32.

19. Joshi C, Russell G, Cheng I-H, Kay M, Pottie K, Alston M et al. A narrative synthesis of the impact of primary health care delivery models for refugees in resettlement countries on access, quality and coordination. Int J Equity Health. 2013;12:88.

20. Wangdahl J, Lytsy P, Martensson L, Westerling R. Health literacy among refugees in Sweden: a cross-sectional study. BMC Public Health. 2014;14:1030.

21. Turner SW, Herlihy J. Working with refugees and asylum seekers. Psychiatry. 2009;8(8):322–4.

22. Clinton-Davis L, Fassil Y. Health and social problems of refugees. Soc Sci Med. 1992;35(4):507–13.

23. Webb E, Ryan AD, O'Hare BAM. The needs of children newly arrived from abroad. Curr Paediatr. 2005;15(4):339–46.

24. van den Heuevel WJ. Health status of refugees from former Yugoslavia: descriptive study of the refugees in the Netherlands. Croat Med J. 1998;39(3):356–60.